LOW GLYCEMIC INDEX DIET COOKBOOK FOR SENIORS 2024

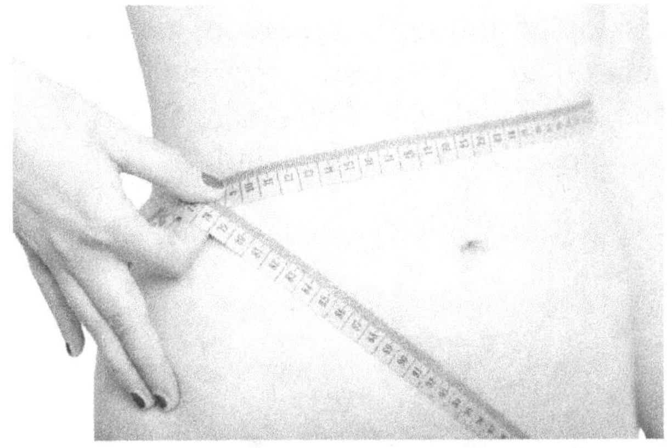

Embark on a Culinary Journey: The Seniors' Delight - A 2024 Cookbook Redefining Health with Low Glycemic Index Recipes, Elevating Flavor, and Nourishing Well-being for a Vibrant Life Ahead!

Felicia O. Pace

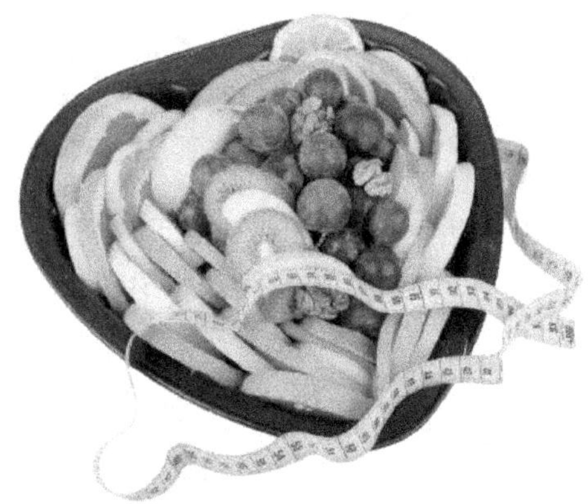

TABLE OF CONTENTS

OTHER BOOKS FROM THE SAME AUTHOUR

LOW GLYCEMIC INDEX FOOD GUIDE CHART 2024

GLYCEMIC INDEX FOOD GUIDE CHART 2024

INTRODUCTION

Welcome to the "Seniors' Low Glycemic Index Diet Cookbook 2024: Nourishing Your Health with Smart Choices." This cookbook is crafted with care and tailored to meet the unique nutritional needs of seniors, providing a wealth of delicious recipes that align with the principles of a low glycemic index (GI) diet. As we age, maintaining a balanced and wholesome diet becomes increasingly crucial for overall well-being, and the low GI approach offers a sensible and healthful way to do so.

Understanding Glycemic Index and Glycemic Load:

The Glycemic Index measures how quickly a carbohydrate-containing food raises blood glucose levels. Foods are ranked on a scale from 0 to 100, with higher values signifying faster digestion and a more rapid increase in blood sugar. The Glycemic Load combines the quantity and quality of carbohydrates, providing a more comprehensive view of a food's impact on blood sugar. In this cookbook, we leverage these principles to guide you toward making mindful choices that contribute to stable blood sugar levels.

Best Low GI Foods to Eat:

Our cookbook places a spotlight on a variety of nutrient-rich, low GI foods that form the foundation of your meals. Whole grains like quinoa and barley, legumes such as lentils and chickpeas, colorful vegetables, lean proteins, and healthy fats are the stars of these recipes. By incorporating these wholesome ingredients, you can enjoy satisfying, flavorful meals that contribute to sustained energy and promote optimal health.

Benefits of a Low Glycemic Index for Seniors:

Blood Sugar Management: For seniors, managing blood sugar levels is paramount. A low GI diet helps stabilize glucose levels, reducing the risk of spikes and crashes, which can be particularly beneficial for those with diabetes or at risk of developing it.

Heart Health: Many low GI foods, such as whole grains and heart-healthy fats, support cardiovascular health. These choices can contribute to lower cholesterol levels and a reduced risk of heart disease, a concern that becomes increasingly prevalent as we age.

Weight Management: Maintaining a healthy weight is essential for overall well-being. The sustained energy provided by low GI foods can aid in weight management, supporting seniors in achieving and sustaining an optimal body weight.

Cognitive Function: A diet rich in low GI foods has been associated with improved cognitive function. For seniors, this is particularly significant, as it may contribute to maintaining mental acuity and reducing the risk of cognitive decline.

Digestive Health: The fiber content in many low GI foods supports digestive health, promoting regular bowel movements and preventing constipation, a common concern for seniors.

This cookbook is your guide to embracing a low GI lifestyle, promoting not only better blood sugar management but also an overall healthier and more vibrant senior life. Let's embark on this flavorful and nutritious journey together!

Low glycemic Snacks and appetizer

1. Greek Yogurt Parfait

Ingredients:
1 cup Greek yogurt
1/4 cup fresh berries (e.g., blueberries, strawberries)
1 tablespoon chopped nuts (e.g., almonds, walnuts)
1 teaspoon honey

Preparation:
1. Layer Greek yogurt in a bowl or glass.

2. Add fresh berries on top.
3. Sprinkle with chopped nuts.
4. Drizzle with honey.

Prep Time: 5 minutes
GI Value: 23
GI Load: 6
Calories: ~200
Sugar Level: 10g

2. Hummus with Veggie Sticks

Ingredients:
1/2 cup hummus
Carrot sticks, cucumber slices, and bell pepper strips
for dipping

Preparation:
1. Place hummus in a bowl.
2. Arrange veggie sticks for dipping.

Prep Time: 10 minutes
GI Value: 6
GI Load: 1
Calories: ~150
Sugar Level: 2g

3. Deviled Eggs with Avocado

Ingredients:
4 hard-boiled eggs
1 ripe avocado
1 tablespoon Greek yogurt
Paprika for garnish
Preparation:
1. Cut eggs in half, remove yolks.

2. Mash yolks with avocado and Greek yogurt.
3. Spoon mixture back into egg whites.
4. Sprinkle it with paprika.

Prep Time: 15 minutes
GI Value: 15
GI Load: 3
Calories: ~180
Sugar Level: 1g

4. Baked Sweet Potato Chips

Ingredients:
2 sweet potatoes, thinly sliced
1 tablespoon olive oil
Sea salt to taste

Preparation:
1. Preheat the oven to 400°F (200°C).
2. Toss sweet potato slices in olive oil and salt.
3. Bake until crispy.

Prep Time: 25 minutes
GI Value: 41
GI Load: 12
Calories: ~120
Sugar Level: 5g

5. Cottage Cheese and Pineapple Skewers

Ingredients:
1 cup low-fat cottage cheese
1 cup fresh pineapple chunks

Preparation:

Alternate threading cottage cheese and pineapple onto skewers.
Prep Time: 10 minutes
GI Value: 15
GI Load: 4
Calories: ~130
Sugar Level: 10g

6. Almond and Chia Seed Pudding

Ingredients:
1/4 cup chia seeds
1 cup unsweetened almond milk
1/2 teaspoon vanilla extract
Stevia for sweetness (optional)

Preparation:
1. Mix chia seeds, almond milk, and vanilla extract.
2. Refrigerate until pudding is consistent.

Prep Time: 5 minutes (+ refrigeration)
GI Value: 1
GI Load: 0
Calories: ~100
Sugar Level: 0g

7. Caprese Salad Skewers

Ingredients:
Cherry tomatoes
Fresh mozzarella balls
Basil leaves
Balsamic glaze for drizzling
Preparation:

Thread a tomato, mozzarella ball, and basil leaf onto skewers.
Drizzle with balsamic glaze.
Prep Time: 10 minutes
GI Value: 15
GI Load: 4
Calories: ~120
Sugar Level: 3g

8. Quinoa and Black Bean Salad

Ingredients:
1 cup cooked quinoa
1/2 cup black beans (canned, drained, and rinsed)
Cherry tomatoes, cucumber, and bell pepper, diced
Olive oil and lemon juice dressing

Preparation:
Mix quinoa, black beans, and diced vegetables.
Toss with olive oil and lemon juice dressing.
Prep Time: 15 minutes
GI Value: 53
GI Load: 13
Calories: ~180
Sugar Level: 2g

9. Sliced Apple with Peanut Butter

Ingredients:
1 apple, thinly sliced
2 tablespoons natural peanut butter

Preparation:

Spread peanut butter on apple slices.
Prep Time: 5 minutes
GI Value: 35
GI Load: 11
Calories: ~160
Sugar Level: 10g

10. Stuffed Bell Peppers with Tuna

Ingredients:
2 bell peppers, halved and deseeded
1 can tuna, drained
1/4 cup diced celery
1 tablespoon olive oil
Salt and pepper to taste

Preparation:
Mix tuna, celery, olive oil, salt, and pepper.
Stuffed bell pepper halves with the mixture.
Prep Time: 20 minutes
GI Value: 0
GI Load: 0
Calories: ~150
Sugar Level: 1g

Low glycemic Desserts and Treats

1. Baked Cinnamon Apples

Ingredients:
2 apples, cored and sliced
1 teaspoon cinnamon
1 tablespoon melted coconut oil
1 tablespoon chopped nuts (optional)

Preparation:
1. Preheat the oven to 350°F (175°C).
2. Toss apples with cinnamon and coconut oil.
3. Bake until tender.
4. Sprinkle with nuts if desired.

Prep Time: 20 minutes
GI Value: 38
GI Load: 10
Calories: ~120
Sugar Level: 10g

2. Chia Seed Pudding with Berries

Ingredients:
1/4 cup chia seeds
1 cup unsweetened almond milk
1/2 cup mixed berries
Stevia for sweetness (optional)

Preparation:
1. Mix chia seeds and almond milk.
2. Refrigerate until pudding is consistent.
3. Top with mixed berries before serving.

Prep Time: 5 minutes (+ refrigeration)

GI Value: 1
GI Load: 0
Calories: ~150
Sugar Level: 2g

3. Dark Chocolate-Covered Strawberries

Ingredients:
1 cup fresh strawberries
2 ounces dark chocolate (70% cocoa or higher)

Preparation:
1. Melt dark chocolate in a microwave or double boiler.
2. Dip strawberries in melted chocolate.
3. Place on parchment paper to cool.

Prep Time: 15 minutes
GI Value: 25
GI Load: 6
Calories: ~100
Sugar Level: 5g

4. Avocado Chocolate Mousse

Ingredients:
2 ripe avocados
1/4 cup cocoa powder
1/4 cup maple syrup
1 teaspoon vanilla extract

Preparation:
1. Blend avocados, cocoa powder, maple syrup, and vanilla until smooth.
2. Chill before serving.

Prep Time: 10 minutes (+ chilling)
GI Value: 15
GI Load: 5
Calories: ~150
Sugar Level: 8g

5. Almond Flour Banana Muffins

Ingredients:
2 ripe bananas, mashed
1 cup almond flour
2 eggs
1 teaspoon baking powder

Preparation:
1. Mix mashed bananas, almond flour, eggs, and baking powder.
2. Pour into muffin cups.
3. Bake until golden brown.

Prep Time: 25 minutes
GI Value: 35
GI Load: 9
Calories: ~120
Sugar Level: 5g

6. Coconut and Lime Sorbet

Ingredients:
2 cups coconut milk
Zest and juice of 2 limes
Stevia for sweetness (optional)

Preparation:
1. Mix coconut milk with lime zest and juice.
2. Freeze in an ice cream maker.
3. Sweeten with stevia if desired.

Prep Time: 15 minutes (+ freezing)
GI Value: 35
GI Load: 9
Calories: ~100
Sugar Level: 2g

7. Pumpkin Chia Seed Pudding

Ingredients:
1/2 cup canned pumpkin puree
1/4 cup chia seeds
1 cup unsweetened almond milk
1/2 teaspoon pumpkin spice

Preparation:
1. Mix pumpkin puree, chia seeds, almond milk, and pumpkin spice.
2. Refrigerate until pudding is consistent.

Prep Time: 5 minutes (+ refrigeration)
GI Value: 1
GI Load: 0
Calories: ~120
Sugar Level: 3g

8. Walnut and Date Energy Bites

Ingredients:
1 cup pitted dates
1/2 cup walnuts
1 tablespoon chia seeds
1/2 teaspoon vanilla extract

Preparation:
Blend dates, walnuts, chia seeds, and vanilla until sticky.
Roll into bite-sized balls.
Prep Time: 15 minutes
GI Value: 42
GI Load: 10
Calories: ~100
Sugar Level: 8g

9. Berry and Yogurt Popsicles

Ingredients:
1 cup mixed berries
1 cup Greek yogurt
Stevia for sweetness (optional)

Preparation:
1. Blend berries and Greek yogurt.
2. Sweeten with stevia if desired.
3. Pour into popsicle molds and freeze.
Prep Time: 10 minutes (+ freezing)
GI Value: 23
GI Load: 6
Calories: ~80
Sugar Level: 6g

10. Cocoa and Almond Butter Protein Balls

Ingredients:
1/2 cup almond butter
1/4 cup cocoa powder
1/4 cup protein powder
1 tablespoon honey

Preparation:
1. Mix almond butter, cocoa powder, protein powder, and honey.
2. Roll into small balls.

Prep Time: 15 minutes
GI Value: 18
GI Load: 5
Calories: ~90
Sugar Level: 4g

Low Glycemic Beverages

1. Green Tea with Lemon

Ingredients:
Green tea bag
Hot water
Slices of fresh lemon

Preparation:
1. Steep the green tea bag in hot water.
2. Add slices of fresh lemon for flavor.

Prep Time: 5 minutes

GI Value: 0
GI Load: 0
Calories: ~5
Sugar Level: 0g

2. Iced Herbal Infusion

Ingredients:
Herbal tea bag (e.g., chamomile, peppermint)
Cold water
Ice cubes
Fresh mint leaves (optional)

Preparation:
1. Steep the herbal tea bag in cold water.
2. Add ice cubes and fresh mint leaves if desired.

Prep Time: 10 minutes
GI Value: 0
GI Load: 0
Calories: ~5
Sugar Level: 0g

3. Sparkling Berry Lemonade

Ingredients:
Sparkling water
Fresh berries (e.g., raspberries, blueberries)
Freshly squeezed lemon juice
Stevia for sweetness (optional)

Preparation:

1. Mix sparkling water, fresh berries, and lemon
    juice.
2. Sweeten with stevia if desired.

Prep Time: 5 minutes
GI Value: 23
GI Load: 6
Calories: ~15
Sugar Level: 3g

4. Cucumber and Mint Infused Water

Ingredients:
Sliced cucumber
Fresh mint leaves
Cold water
Ice cubes

Preparation:
1. Combine sliced cucumber and mint leaves in
    cold water.
2. Add ice cubes and let it infuse.

Prep Time: 5 minutes
GI Value: 0
GI Load: 0
Calories: ~5
Sugar Level: 0g

5. Almond Milk Smoothie

Ingredients:
1 cup unsweetened almond milk
1/2 cup frozen berries
1 tablespoon chia seeds
Stevia for sweetness (optional)

Preparation:
1. Blend almond milk, frozen berries, and chia seeds.
2. Sweeten with stevia if desired.

Prep Time: 5 minutes
GI Value: 35
GI Load: 9
Calories: ~80
Sugar Level: 4g

6. Tomato and Basil Juice

Ingredients:
1 cup tomato juice (low sodium)
Fresh basil leaves
Dash of black pepper

Preparation:
1. Mix tomato juice with torn basil leaves.
2. Add a dash of black pepper for flavor.

Prep Time: 5 minutes
GI Value: 38
GI Load: 10
Calories: ~40
Sugar Level: 8g

7. Coconut Water and Pineapple Cooler

Ingredients:
1 cup coconut water
1/2 cup fresh pineapple chunks
Ice cubes

Preparation:
1. Combine coconut water and pineapple chunks.
2. Add ice cubes and stir.

Prep Time: 5 minutes
GI Value: 3
GI Load: 1
Calories: ~50
Sugar Level: 9g

8. Ginger Turmeric Tea

Ingredients:
Ginger root, grated
Turmeric powder
Hot water
Lemon wedge

Preparation:
1. Steep grated ginger and turmeric powder in hot water.
2. Garnish with a lemon wedge.

Prep Time: 10 minutes
GI Value: 0
GI Load: 0
Calories: ~10
Sugar Level: 0g

9. Peach and Mint Iced Tea

Ingredients:
Peach tea bag
Cold water
Fresh mint leaves
Ice cubes

Preparation:
Steep peach tea bag in cold water.
Add fresh mint leaves and ice cubes.
Prep Time: 10 minutes
GI Value: 0
GI Load: 0
Calories: ~5
Sugar Level: 0g

10. Berry and Avocado Smoothie

Ingredients:
1/2 cup mixed berries (fresh or frozen)
1/4 avocado
1 cup unsweetened almond milk
Stevia for sweetness (optional)

Preparation:
Blend berries, avocado, and almond milk.
Sweeten with stevia if desired.
Prep Time: 5 minutes
GI Value: 35
GI Load: 9
Calories: ~100
Sugar Level: 4g

Low Glycemic Fruits

1. Berries Salad with Mint

Ingredients:
1 cup mixed berries (e.g., blueberries, raspberries, strawberries)
Fresh mint leaves
1 teaspoon lemon juice

Preparation:
1. Wash and mix the berries in a bowl.
2. Sprinkle with fresh mint leaves and drizzle lemon juice.

Prep Time: 5 minutes
GI Value: 25
GI Load: 6
Calories: ~50
Sugar Level: 5g

2. Apple Slices with Almond Butter

Ingredients:
1 apple, sliced
2 tablespoons almond butter

Preparation:
1. Arrange apple slices on a plate.
2. Dip slices in almond butter before eating.

Prep Time: 5 minutes
GI Value: 36
GI Load: 6
Calories: ~120
Sugar Level: 10g

3. Peach and Yogurt Parfait

Ingredients:
1 ripe peach, sliced
1/2 cup Greek yogurt
1 tablespoon chopped almonds

Preparation:
1. Layer peach slices and Greek yogurt in a glass.
2. Top with chopped almonds.

Prep Time: 7 minutes
GI Value: 28
GI Load: 7
Calories: ~100
Sugar Level: 8g

4. Pear and Cheese Platter

Ingredients:
1 pear, sliced
1 ounce of goat cheese or brie
Handful of walnuts

Preparation:
1. Arrange pear slices on a plate.
2. Pair with small portions of cheese and walnuts.

Prep Time: 7 minutes
GI Value: 38
GI Load: 10
Calories: ~120
Sugar Level: 8g

5. Plum and Cottage Cheese Bowl

Ingredients:
2 plums, sliced
1/2 cup low-fat cottage cheese
1 tablespoon flax seeds (optional)

Preparation:
1. Mix plum slices with cottage cheese in a bowl.
2. Sprinkle with flax seeds if desired.

Prep Time: 5 minutes
GI Value: 39
GI Load: 9
Calories: ~100
Sugar Level: 10g

6. Kiwi and Pineapple Skewers

Ingredients:
Kiwi, peeled and sliced
Pineapple chunks

Preparation:
Thread kiwi slices and pineapple chunks onto skewers.
Prep Time: 7 minutes
GI Value: 47
GI Load: 12
Calories: ~80
Sugar Level: 8g

7. Grapefruit Segments with Mint

Ingredients:
1 grapefruit, segmented
Fresh mint leaves

Preparation:
1. Segment the grapefruit and arrange on a plate.
2. Garnish with fresh mint leaves.

Prep Time: 7 minutes
GI Value: 25
GI Load: 6
Calories: ~50
Sugar Level: 8g

8. Melon and Prosciutto Bites

Ingredients:
Melon cubes (e.g., cantaloupe, honeydew)
Thin slices of prosciutto

Preparation:
Wrap melon cubes with prosciutto slices.
Prep Time: 10 minutes
GI Value: 60
GI Load: 14
Calories: ~70
Sugar Level: 8g

9. Cherry Tomato and Mozzarella Skewers

Ingredients:
Cherry tomatoes
Mini mozzarella balls
Fresh basil leaves

Preparation:
Thread cherry tomatoes, mini mozzarella balls, and basil leaves onto skewers.
Prep Time: 8 minutes
GI Value: 15
GI Load: 4
Calories: ~60
Sugar Level: 4g

10. Orange and Walnut Salad

Ingredients:
1 orange, peeled and segmented
Mixed salad greens
1 tablespoon chopped walnuts

Preparation:
Toss orange segments with mixed salad greens.
Sprinkle with chopped walnuts.
Prep Time: 7 minutes
GI Value: 40
GI Load: 10
Calories: ~70
Sugar Level: 9g

Low glycemic Vegetables

1. Roasted Brussels Sprouts

Ingredients:
Brussels sprouts, halved
Olive oil
Garlic powder
Salt and pepper

Preparation:
1. Toss Brussels sprouts with olive oil, garlic powder, salt, and pepper.
2. Roast in the oven until golden brown.

Prep Time: 25 minutes
GI Value: 15
GI Load: 4
Caories: ~80
Sugar Level: 2g

2. Steamed Asparagus with Lemon

Ingredients:
Fresh asparagus spears
Lemon zest
Olive oil
Salt

Preparation:
Steam asparagus until tender.
Drizzle with olive oil, sprinkle lemon zest, and add a pinch of salt.

Prep Time: 15 minutes

GI Value: 15
GI Load: 2
Calories: ~30
Sugar Level: 2g

3. Sauteed Spinach with Garlic

Ingredients:
Fresh spinach leaves
Garlic, minced
Olive oil
Lemon juice

Preparation:
1. Saute garlic in olive oil until fragrant.
2. Add spinach and cook until wilted.
3. Finish with a squeeze of lemon juice.

Prep Time: 10 minutes
GI Value: 15
GI Load: 2
Calories: ~20
Sugar Level: 0g

4. Grilled Zucchini with Herbs

Ingredients:
Zucchini, sliced
Olive oil
Fresh herbs (rosemary, thyme)
Salt and pepper

Preparation:
1. Toss zucchini with olive oil, fresh herbs, salt, and pepper.
2. Grill until tender.

Prep Time: 20 minutes
GI Value: 15
GI Load: 2
Calories: ~30
Sugar Level: 2g

5. Baked Cauliflower Bites

Ingredients:
Cauliflower florets
Paprika
Parmesan cheese
Olive oil

1. **Preparation:**
2. Toss cauliflower with olive oil, paprika, and Parmesan.
3. Bake until golden brown.

Prep Time: 30 minutes
GI Value: 15
GI Load: 2
Calories: ~40
Sugar Level: 2g

6. Stir-Fried Broccoli with Ginger

Ingredients:
Broccoli florets

Ginger, minced
Soy sauce
Sesame oil

Preparation:
1. Stir-fry broccoli with minced ginger in sesame oil.
2. Add soy sauce for flavor.

Prep Time: 15 minutes
GI Value: 10
GI Load: 2
Calories: ~30
Sugar Level: 2g

7. Cabbage and Carrot Slaw

Ingredients:
Shredded cabbage and carrots
Greek yogurt
Dijon mustard
Apple cider vinegar

Preparation:
1. Mix shredded cabbage and carrots.
2. Combine Greek yogurt, Dijon mustard, and apple cider vinegar for dressing.

Prep Time: 15 minutes
GI Value: 10
GI Load: 2
Calories: ~40
Sugar Level: 3g

8. Roasted Eggplant with Tahini

Ingredients:
Eggplant, sliced
Olive oil
Tahini
Lemon juice

Preparation:
1. Brush eggplant slices with olive oil and roast until tender.
2. Drizzle with tahini and lemon juice.

Prep Time: 30 minutes
GI Value: 15
GI Load: 2
Calories: ~50
Sugar Level: 2g

9. Cucumber and Avocado Salad

Ingredients:
Cucumber, sliced
Avocado, diced
Red onion, thinly sliced
Olive oil and balsamic vinegar

Preparation:
1. Combine cucumber, avocado, and red onion.
2. Dress with olive oil and balsamic vinegar.

Prep Time: 10 minutes
GI Value: 15
GI Load: 2

Calories: ~60
Sugar Level: 2g

10. Sautéed Mushrooms with Thyme

Ingredients:
Mushrooms, sliced
Garlic, minced
Fresh thyme
Olive oil

Preparation:
1. Sauté mushrooms and garlic in olive oil.
2. Add fresh thyme for flavor.

Prep Time: 15 minutes
GI Value: 10
GI Load: 2
Calories: ~20
Sugar Level: 2g

Low glycemic legumes and pulse

1. Lentil and Vegetable Soup

Ingredients:
1 cup dry lentils
Assorted vegetables (carrots, celery, onions)
Low-sodium vegetable broth
Garlic, minced
Olive oil
Herbs and spices (thyme, bay leaves)

Preparation:

1. Sauté garlic, onions, and vegetables in olive oil.
2. Add lentils, vegetable broth, and herbs.
3. Simmer until lentils are tender.

Prep Time: 40 minutes
GI Value: 29
GI Load: 9
Calories: ~200
Sugar Level: 4g

2. Chickpea and Spinach Salad

Ingredients:
1 can chickpeas, drained and rinsed
Fresh spinach leaves
Cherry tomatoes, halved
Feta cheese
Olive oil and balsamic vinegar

Preparation:
1. Combine chickpeas, spinach, tomatoes, and feta.
2. Drizzle with olive oil and balsamic vinegar.

Prep Time: 15 minutes
GI Value: 28
GI Load: 9
Calories: ~250
Sugar Level: 3g

3. Black Bean and Avocado Wrap

Ingredients:
1 can black beans, drained and rinsed
Whole-grain wraps

Avocado, sliced
Salsa
Shredded lettuce

Preparation:
1. Mash black beans and spread on wraps.
2. Layer with avocado slices, salsa, and shredded lettuce.
3. Roll into a wrap.

Prep Time: 15 minutes
GI Value: 30
GI Load: 9
Calories: ~300
Sugar Level: 2g

4. Split Pea and Ham Soup

Ingredients:
1 cup split peas
Ham, diced
Carrots, celery, onions
Low-sodium chicken broth
Garlic, minced
Herbs (bay leaves, thyme)

Preparation:
1. Sauté garlic, onions, and vegetables.
2. Add split peas, ham, and chicken broth.
3. Simmer until peas are soft.

Prep Time: 50 minutes
GI Value: 32
GI Load: 10
Calories: ~220
Sugar Level: 4g

5. Edamame and Quinoa Salad

Ingredients:
Edamame beans, cooked
Quinoa, cooked
Cherry tomatoes, halved
Cucumber, diced
Feta cheese
Lemon vinaigrette

Preparation:
1. Combine edamame, quinoa, tomatoes, cucumber, and feta.
2. Drizzle with lemon vinaigrette.

Prep Time: 20 minutes
GI Value: 35
GI Load: 10
Calories: ~280
Sugar Level: 4g

6. Adzuki Bean and Vegetable Stir-Fry

Ingredients:
1 cup adzuki beans, cooked
Mixed vegetables (broccoli, bell peppers, snap peas)
Low-sodium soy sauce
Sesame oil
Ginger, minced

Preparation:

1.   Stir-fry vegetables and ginger in sesame oil.
2.   Add cooked adzuki beans and soy sauce.

Prep Time: 20 minutes

GI Value: 42
GI Load: 12
Calories: ~220
Sugar Level: 3g

7. Pinto Bean and Corn Salsa

Ingredients:
1 can pinto beans, drained and rinsed
Corn kernels
Red onion, finely chopped
Cilantro, chopped
Lime juice
Chili powder

Preparation:
Mix pinto beans, corn, red onion, and cilantro.
Dress with lime juice and sprinkle chili powder.
Prep Time: 15 minutes
GI Value: 45
GI Load: 12
Calories: ~180
Sugar Level: 3g

8. Mung Bean Salad with Cumin Dressing

Ingredients:
1 cup mung beans, cooked

Cherry tomatoes, halved
Red bell pepper, diced
Red onion, finely chopped
Cumin dressing (olive oil, cumin, lemon juice)

Preparation:
1. Combine cooked mung beans, tomatoes, bell pepper, and red onion.
2. Drizzle with cumin dressing.

Prep Time: 25 minutes
GI Value: 25
GI Load: 7
Calories: ~200
Sugar Level: 4g

9. White Bean and Rosemary Dip

Ingredients:
1 can white beans, drained and rinsed
Fresh rosemary, chopped
Garlic, minced
Olive oil
Lemon juice

Preparation:
Blend white beans, rosemary, garlic, olive oil, and lemon juice.
Serve as a dip with veggies.
Prep Time: 10 minutes
GI Value: 30
GI Load: 9
Calories: ~120
Sugar Level: 1g

10. Black-eyed Pea and Brown Rice Bowl

Ingredients:
1 cup black-eyed peas, cooked
Brown rice, cooked
Sautéed spinach and garlic
Cherry tomatoes, halved
Lemon tahini dressing

Preparation:
1. Layer black-eyed peas, brown rice, sautéed spinach, and tomatoes.
2. Drizzle with lemon tahini dressing.

Prep Time: 30 minutes
GI Value: 40
GI Load: 11
Calories: ~250
Sugar Level: 3g

Low glycemic Whole grains

1. Quinoa Salad with Vegetables

Ingredients:
1 cup quinoa, rinsed
Mixed vegetables (bell peppers, cucumber, cherry tomatoes)

Olive oil and lemon vinaigrette
Fresh herbs (parsley, mint)

Preparation:
1. Cook quinoa according to package instructions.
2. Mix quinoa with chopped vegetables.
3. Drizzle with olive oil and lemon vinaigrette, and garnish with fresh herbs.

Prep Time: 20 minutes
GI Value: 53
GI Load: 13
Calories: ~250
Sugar Level: 2g

2. Brown Rice and Lentil Pilaf

Ingredients:
1 cup brown rice
1/2 cup lentils
Mixed vegetables (carrots, peas, onions)
Low-sodium vegetable broth
Olive oil
Cumin and coriander

Preparation:
1. Sauté vegetables in olive oil.
2. Add brown rice, lentils, vegetable broth, and spices. Simmer until cooked.

Prep Time: 40 minutes
GI Value: 50
GI Load: 12

Calories: ~280
Sugar Level: 3g

3. Barley and Mushroom Risotto

Ingredients:
1 cup barley
Mushrooms, sliced
Onion, finely chopped
Low-sodium vegetable broth
Parmesan cheese
Thyme and garlic

Preparation:
Sauté mushrooms and onions in olive oil.
Add barley, vegetable broth, thyme, and garlic. Cook
until creamy.
Stir in Parmesan cheese.
Prep Time: 45 minutes
GI Value: 28
GI Load: 7
Calories: ~300
Sugar Level: 3g

4. Oatmeal with Berries and Almonds

Ingredients:
1/2 cup rolled oats
Mixed berries (blueberries, strawberries)
Almonds, chopped
Cinnamon and nutmeg
Almond milk

Preparation:

1. Cook oats with almond milk, cinnamon, and nutmeg.
2. Top with mixed berries and chopped almonds.

Prep Time: 10 minutes
GI Value: 55
GI Load: 13
Calories: ~200
Sugar Level: 4g

5. Buckwheat Pancakes with Greek Yogurt

Ingredients:
1 cup buckwheat flour
Baking powder
Eggs
Greek yogurt
Fresh berries

Preparation:

1. Mix buckwheat flour, baking powder, and eggs to form a batter.
2. Cook pancakes and serve with Greek yogurt and fresh berries.

Prep Time: 25 minutes
GI Value: 54

GI Load: 13
Calories: ~250
Sugar Level: 5g

6. Millet and Vegetable Stir-Fry

Ingredients:
1 cup millet, cooked
Mixed vegetables (broccoli, carrots, bell peppers)
Tofu or chicken
Soy sauce
Sesame oil
Ginger and garlic

Preparation:
1. Stir-fry tofu or chicken with vegetables, ginger, and garlic.
2. Add cooked millet, soy sauce, and sesame oil.

Prep Time: 30 minutes
GI Value: 71
GI Load: 15
Calories: ~300
Sugar Level: 2g

7. Whole Wheat Pasta with Tomato and Basil

Ingredients:
Whole wheat pasta
Tomatoes, diced
Fresh basil, chopped

Olive oil
Garlic, minced
Parmesan cheese

Preparation:
1. Cook whole wheat pasta according to package instructions.
2. Sauté garlic in olive oil, add tomatoes and basil. Toss with cooked pasta.
3. Sprinkle with Parmesan cheese.

Prep Time: 25 minutes
GI Value: 37
GI Load: 9
Calories: ~300
Sugar Level: 4g

8. Spelt and Vegetable Casserole

Ingredients:
1 cup spelt, cooked
Mixed vegetables (zucchini, bell peppers, cherry tomatoes)
Feta cheese
Olive oil
Italian herbs

Preparation:
1. Mix cooked spelt with roasted vegetables and feta cheese.
2. Drizzle with olive oil and sprinkle Italian herbs.

Prep Time: 30 minutes

GI Value: 54
GI Load: 13
Calories: ~250
Sugar Level: 3g

9. Wild Rice and Cranberry Salad

Ingredients:
1 cup wild rice, cooked
Dried cranberries
Pecans, chopped
Orange vinaigrette
Fresh parsley

Preparation:
1. Mix cooked wild rice with cranberries and pecans.
2. Drizzle with orange vinaigrette and garnish with fresh parsley.

Prep Time: 35 minutes
GI Value: 57
GI Load: 14
Calories: ~280
Sugar Level: 6g

10. Amaranth Porridge with Mango

Ingredients:
1/2 cup amaranth, cooked
Mango, diced
Coconut milk
Honey or maple syrup
Chia seeds

Preparation:
1. Cook amaranth in coconut milk until creamy.
2. Top with diced mango, chia seeds, and a drizzle of honey or maple syrup.

Prep Time: 25 minutes

GI Value: 65
GI Load: 15
Calories: ~250
Sugar Level: 8g

Low glycemic Dairy and Dairy Alternative

1. Greek Yogurt Parfait with Berries

Ingredients:
Greek yogurt (unsweetened)
Mixed berries (blueberries, strawberries)
Nuts (almonds or walnuts)
Drizzle of honey (optional)

Preparation:
1. Layer Greek yogurt with mixed berries in a glass.
2. Top with nuts and a drizzle of honey if desired.

Prep Time: 5 minutes
GI Value: 30
GI Load: 6
Calories: ~150

Sugar Level: 5g

2. Almond Milk Chia Pudding

Ingredients:
Almond milk (unsweetened)
Chia seeds
Vanilla extract
Fresh berries for topping

Preparation:
1. Mix chia seeds with almond milk and vanilla extract.
2. Refrigerate overnight or until the pudding thickens.
3. Top with fresh berries before serving.

Prep Time: 10 minutes (+ chilling time)
GI Value: 1
GI Load: 0
Calories: ~120
Sugar Level: 1g

3. Cottage Cheese with Pineapple

Ingredients:
Low-fat cottage cheese
Fresh pineapple chunks

Preparation:
Serve a portion of cottage cheese.

Top with fresh pineapple chunks.
Prep Time: 5 minutes
GI Value: 10
GI Load: 2
Calories: ~120
Sugar Level: 8g

4. Coconut Milk Smoothie

Ingredients:
Coconut milk (unsweetened)
Spinach
Banana
Protein powder (optional)

Preparation:
1. Blend coconut milk, spinach, banana, and protein powder until smooth.
2. Pour into a glass and enjoy.

Prep Time: 5 minutes
GI Value: 20
GI Load: 5
Calories: ~200
Sugar Level: 7g

5. Feta and Cucumber Salad

Ingredients:
Feta cheese
Cucumber, sliced
Cherry tomatoes, halved
Olive oil and balsamic vinegar

Preparation:

1. Combine feta, cucumber, and cherry tomatoes in a bowl.
2. Drizzle with olive oil and balsamic vinegar.

Prep Time: 10 minutes
GI Value: 0 (for feta)
GI Load: 0
Calories: ~150
Sugar Level: 3g

6. Low-Fat Yogurt with Mango Slices

Ingredients:
Low-fat yogurt (unsweetened)
Fresh mango slices

Preparation:
1. Serve a portion of low-fat yogurt.
2. Top with fresh mango slices.

Prep Time: 5 minutes
GI Value: 30
GI Load: 6
Calories: ~120
Sugar Level: 12g

7. Cashew Milk Rice Pudding

Ingredients:
Cashew milk (unsweetened)
Arborio rice
Cinnamon
Raisins (optional)

Preparation:
Cook Arborio rice in cashew milk until creamy.

Stir in cinnamon and add raisins if desired.
Prep Time: 40 minutes
GI Value: 30
GI Load: 7
Calories: ~180
Sugar Level: 6g

8. Mozzarella and Tomato Caprese Salad

Ingredients:
Fresh mozzarella balls
Cherry tomatoes, halved
Fresh basil leaves
Balsamic glaze

Preparation:
1. Arrange mozzarella balls and cherry tomatoes on a plate.
2. Garnish with fresh basil leaves and drizzle with balsamic glaze.

Prep Time: 10 minutes
GI Value: 0 (for mozzarella)
GI Load: 0
Calories: ~200
Sugar Level: 2g

9. Soy Milk Green Tea Smoothie

Ingredients:
Unsweetened soy milk
Green tea (cooled)
Banana

Spinach
Ice cubes

Preparation:
1. Blend soy milk, green tea, banana, spinach, and ice cubes until smooth.
2. Pour into a glass and enjoy.

Prep Time: 8 minutes
GI Value: 15
GI Load: 4
Calories: ~150
Sugar Level: 6g

10. Ricotta and Berry Parfait

Ingredients:
Ricotta cheese
Mixed berries (strawberries, blueberries)
Honey

Preparation:
1. Layer ricotta with mixed berries in a glass.
2. Drizzle with honey.

Prep Time: 7 minutes
GI Value: 10
GI Load: 2
Calories: ~150
Sugar Level: 8g

Low glycemic Nuts and Seed

1. Almond and Chia Seed Pudding

Ingredients:
Almonds (blanched and sliced)
Chia seeds
Unsweetened almond milk
Vanilla extract
Fresh berries for topping

Preparation:
1. Blend almonds and almond milk until smooth.
2. Mix almond milk blend with chia seeds and vanilla extract.
3. Refrigerate overnight.
4. Top with fresh berries before serving.

Prep Time: 10 minutes (+ chilling time)
GI Value: 0 (for chia seeds)
GI Load: 0
Calories: ~200
Sugar Level: 2g

2. Pumpkin Seed Trail Mix

Ingredients:
Pumpkin seeds (pepitas)
Almonds
Walnuts
Dried cranberries
Dark chocolate chunks (70% cocoa)

Preparation:
1. Mix pumpkin seeds, almonds, walnuts, dried cranberries, and dark chocolate chunks.
2. Portion into snack-sized servings.

Prep Time: 5 minutes
GI Value: 15
GI Load: 4
Calories: ~200
Sugar Level: 5g

3. Walnut and Blueberry Smoothie

Ingredients:
Walnuts
Blueberries (fresh or frozen)
Greek yogurt (unsweetened)
Almond milk
Honey (optional)

Preparation:
1. Blend walnuts, blueberries, Greek yogurt, and almond milk until smooth.
2. Sweeten with honey if desired.

Prep Time: 5 minutes
GI Value: 15
GI Load: 4
Calories: ~250
Sugar Level: 8g

4. Cashew and Coconut Energy Bites

Ingredients:

Cashews
Shredded coconut (unsweetened)
Dates (pitted)
Vanilla extract
Sea salt

Preparation:
1. Blend cashews, shredded coconut, dates, vanilla extract, and a pinch of sea salt.
2. Roll into bite-sized balls.

Prep Time: 15 minutes

GI Value: 23
GI Load: 6
Calories: ~150
Sugar Level: 10g

5. Sunflower Seed and Kale Salad

Ingredients:
Sunflower seeds
Kale, finely chopped
Cherry tomatoes, halved
Feta cheese
Olive oil and balsamic vinegar

Preparation:
1. Toast sunflower seeds.
2. Toss kale, cherry tomatoes, and feta.
3. Drizzle with olive oil and balsamic vinegar.

Prep Time: 10 minutes
GI Value: 10
GI Load: 2
Calories: ~200

Sugar Level: 3g

6. Hazelnut and Raspberry Yogurt Parfait

Ingredients:
Hazelnuts, chopped
Greek yogurt (unsweetened)
Fresh raspberries
Honey

Preparation:
1. Layer hazelnuts with Greek yogurt and fresh raspberries in a glass.
2. Drizzle with honey.

Prep Time: 7 minutes
GI Value: 15
GI Load: 3
Calories: ~180
Sugar Level: 8g

7. Chia Seed and Walnut Oatmeal

Ingredients:
Walnuts, chopped
Rolled oats
Chia seeds
Almond milk
Cinnamon and nutmeg

Preparation:

1. Combine rolled oats, chia seeds, and almond milk in a pot.
2. Cook until the oats are soft.
3. Top with chopped walnuts, cinnamon, and nutmeg.

Prep Time: 15 minutes
GI Value: 30
GI Load: 7
Calories: ~250
Sugar Level: 4g

8. Pistachio and Avocado Salad

Ingredients:
Pistachios, shelled
Avocado, diced
Mixed greens
Feta cheese
Lemon vinaigrette

Preparation:
1. Toast pistachios.
2. Combine pistachios, avocado, mixed greens, and feta.
3. Dress with lemon vinaigrette.

Prep Time: 12 minutes
GI Value: 15
GI Load: 4
Calories: ~220
Sugar Level: 3g

9. Flaxseed and Banana Smoothie Bowl

Ingredients:
Flaxseeds
Banana
Spinach
Almond milk
Toppings: Sliced banana, chia seeds, shredded coconut

Preparation:
1. Blend flaxseeds, banana, spinach, and almond milk until smooth.
2. Pour into a bowl and add toppings.

Prep Time: 8 minutes
GI Value: 0 (for flaxseeds)
GI Load: 0
Calories: ~220
Sugar Level: 9g

10. Macadamia Nut and Pineapple Snack

Ingredients:
Macadamia nuts
Fresh pineapple chunks

Preparation:
Combine macadamia nuts and fresh pineapple chunks in a bowl.
Prep Time: 5 minutes
GI Value: 15
GI Load: 2

Calories: ~180
Sugar Level: 8g

Low glycemic Fats and Oil

1. Extra Virgin Olive Oil and Herb Marinade

Ingredients:
Extra virgin olive oil
Fresh herbs (rosemary, thyme, oregano)
Garlic, minced
Lemon juice
Salt and pepper to taste

Preparation:
1. Mix olive oil, minced garlic, fresh herbs, lemon juice, salt, and pepper in a bowl.
2. Use as a marinade for grilled vegetables or lean proteins.

Prep Time: 10 minutes

Calories: ~120 per tablespoon
Sugar Level: 0g

2. Avocado and Lime Dressing

Ingredients:
Ripe avocado
Lime juice
Olive oil
Salt and cayenne pepper to taste

Preparation:
1. Mash the avocado and mix it with lime juice.
2. Add olive oil, salt, and cayenne pepper to create a creamy dressing.
3. Use on salads or as a dip for vegetables.

Prep Time: 5 minutes
Calories: ~90 per tablespoon
Sugar Level: 0g

3. Coconut Oil and Almond Butter Smoothie

Ingredients:
Coconut oil (unrefined)
Almond butter (unsweetened)
Coconut milk (unsweetened)
Chia seeds
Ice cubes

Preparation:
1. Blend coconut oil, almond butter, coconut milk, and chia seeds until smooth.

2.   Add ice cubes for a refreshing smoothie.

Prep Time: 5 minutes

Calories: ~120 per tablespoon of coconut oil

Sugar Level: 1g (from almond butter)

4. Walnut and Flaxseed Pesto

Ingredients:

Walnuts

Flaxseeds

Fresh basil

Garlic, minced

Parmesan cheese (optional)

Extra virgin olive oil

Salt and pepper to taste

Preparation:

1.   Blend walnuts, flaxseeds, basil, garlic, and Parmesan cheese (if using).
2.   Slowly add olive oil while blending until you achieve a smooth pesto.
3.   Season with salt and pepper to taste.
4.   Use as a sauce for whole-grain pasta or as a spread.

Prep Time: 15 minutes

Calories: ~120 per tablespoon

Sugar Level: 0g

5. MCT Oil and Berry Smoothie

Ingredients:

MCT (Medium-Chain Triglyceride) oil

Mixed berries (strawberries, blueberries)

Greek yogurt (unsweetened)
Almond milk (unsweetened)

Preparation:
1. Blend MCT oil, mixed berries, Greek yogurt, and almond milk until smooth.
2. Serve as a nutrient-dense smoothie.

Prep Time: 5 minutes
Calories: ~120 per tablespoon of MCT oil
Sugar Level: 8g (from berries and yogurt)

Low glycemic Seafood

1. Grilled Lemon Garlic Salmon

Ingredients:
Salmon fillets
Fresh lemon juice
Garlic, minced
Olive oil
Salt and pepper to taste

Preparation:
1. Marinate salmon in lemon juice, minced garlic, olive oil, salt, and pepper for 30 minutes.
2. Grill until salmon is cooked through.

Prep Time: 20 minutes (including marination)
Calories: ~200 per 3-ounce serving
Sugar Level: 0g

2. Baked Herb Crusted Cod

Ingredients:
Cod fillets
Fresh herbs (parsley, dill, thyme)
Whole wheat breadcrumbs
Olive oil
Lemon zest
Salt and pepper to taste

Preparation:
1. Mix fresh herbs, breadcrumbs, olive oil, lemon zest, salt, and pepper.
2. Coat cod fillets with the herb mixture.
3. Bake until the fish is flaky.

Prep Time: 25 minutes
Calories: ~150 per 3-ounce serving
Sugar Level: 0g

3. Shrimp and Vegetable Stir-Fry

Ingredients:
Shrimp, peeled and deveined
Mixed vegetables (broccoli, bell peppers, snap peas)
Low-sodium soy sauce
Ginger and garlic, minced
Sesame oil

Preparation:

1. Stir-fry shrimp, mixed vegetables, ginger, and garlic in sesame oil.
2. Add low-sodium soy sauce and cook until the shrimp are pink.

Prep Time: 15 minutes
Calories: ~120 per 3-ounce serving
Sugar Level: 2g

4. Seared Tuna Salad

Ingredients:
Ahi tuna steaks
Mixed salad greens
Cherry tomatoes, halved
Cucumber, sliced
Balsamic vinaigrette

Preparation:
1. Season tuna steaks with salt and pepper.
2. Sear tuna in a hot pan for 1-2 minutes per side.
3. Slice tuna and serve on a bed of mixed greens, tomatoes, and cucumber.
4. Drizzle with balsamic vinaigrette.

Prep Time: 10 minutes
Calories: ~150 per 3-ounce serving
Sugar Level: 3g

5. Broiled Lemon Herb Scallops

Ingredients:
Scallops

Fresh lemon juice
Fresh herbs (thyme, rosemary)
Olive oil
Garlic, minced
Paprika
Salt and pepper to taste

Preparation:
1. Marinate scallops in lemon juice, herbs, olive oil, minced garlic, paprika, salt, and pepper.
2. Broil until scallops are opaque and lightly browned.

Prep Time: 15 minutes (including marination)
Calories: ~100 per 3-ounce serving
Sugar Level: 1g

Low glycemic Herbs and Spices

1. Basil Pesto
Ingredients:
Fresh basil leaves
Pine nuts
Parmesan cheese (optional)
Garlic, minced
Extra virgin olive oil
Salt and pepper to taste

Preparation:
1. Blend basil, pine nuts, Parmesan (if using), and minced garlic in a food processor.

2. Slowly add olive oil while blending until smooth.
3. Season with salt and pepper.

Prep Time: 10 minutes
Calories: ~80 per tablespoon
Sugar Level: 0g

2. Turmeric Roasted Cauliflower

Ingredients:
Cauliflower florets
Turmeric powder
Olive oil
Cumin
Garlic powder
Salt and pepper to taste

Preparation:
1. Toss cauliflower with turmeric, olive oil, cumin, garlic powder, salt, and pepper.
2. Roast until the cauliflower is golden brown.

Prep Time: 20 minutes
Calories: ~50 per cup (cooked)
Sugar Level: 2g

3. Cilantro Lime Quinoa

Ingredients:
Quinoa, rinsed
Fresh cilantro, chopped
Lime juice

Olive oil
Salt and pepper to taste

Preparation:
Cook quinoa according to package instructions.
Mix with chopped cilantro, lime juice, olive oil, salt,
and pepper.
Prep Time: 15 minutes
Calories: ~120 per cup (cooked)
Sugar Level: 0g

4. Rosemary Garlic Roasted Chicken

Ingredients:
Chicken thighs or breasts
Fresh rosemary, chopped
Garlic, minced
Lemon zest
Olive oil
Salt and pepper to taste
Preparation:
Mix rosemary, minced garlic, lemon zest, olive oil,
salt, and pepper.
Coat chicken with the herb mixture and roast until
cooked through.
Prep Time: 30 minutes
Calories: ~200 per 3-ounce serving
Sugar Level: 0g

5. Chili-Lime Grilled Shrimp

Ingredients:
Shrimp, peeled and deveined
Chili powder

Lime juice
Olive oil
Cilantro, chopped
Salt and pepper to taste

Preparation:
1. Marinate shrimp in chili powder, lime juice, olive oil, chopped cilantro, salt, and pepper.
2. Grill until shrimp are opaque.

Prep Time: 15 minutes (including marination)
Calories: ~100 per 3-ounce serving
Sugar Level: 0g

Low glycemic Breakfast Recipes

1. Greek Yogurt with Berries and Almonds

Ingredients:
Greek yogurt (unsweetened)
Mixed berries (blueberries, strawberries)
Almonds (sliced)
Drizzle of honey (optional)

Preparation:

1. Spoon Greek yogurt into a bowl.
2. Top with mixed berries and sliced almonds.
3. Drizzle with honey if desired.

Prep Time: 5 minutes
GI Value: 30
GI Load: 6
Calories: ~200
Sugar Level: 10g

2. Avocado and Tomato Omelette

Ingredients:
Eggs (whisked)
Avocado (sliced)
Cherry tomatoes (halved)
Fresh basil (chopped)
Salt and pepper to taste

Preparation:
1. Make an omelette with whisked eggs.
2. Fill with sliced avocado, cherry tomatoes, and fresh basil.
3. Season with salt and pepper.

Prep Time: 10 minutes
GI Value: 0 (for eggs)
GI Load: 0
Calories: ~250
Sugar Level: 2g

3. Chia Seed Pudding with Almond Milk

Ingredients:
Chia seeds
Almond milk (unsweetened)

Vanilla extract
Fresh berries for topping

Preparation:
1. Mix chia seeds with almond milk and vanilla extract.
2. Refrigerate until the pudding thickens.
3. Top with fresh berries before serving.

Prep Time: 5 minutes (+ chilling time)
GI Value: 1
GI Load: 0
Calories: ~150
Sugar Level: 1g

4. Whole Grain Toast with Smashed Avocado

Ingredients:
Whole grain bread (toasted)
Avocado (smashed)
Cherry tomatoes (sliced)
Sprinkle of sea salt and black pepper
Preparation:
1. Toast whole grain bread.
2. Spread smashed avocado on the toast.
3. Top with sliced cherry tomatoes and season with sea salt and black pepper.

Prep Time: 7 minutes
GI Value: 30 (approximate for whole grain bread)
GI Load: 10
Calories: ~200
Sugar Level: 2g

5. Spinach and Feta Frittata

Ingredients:
Eggs (whisked)
Fresh spinach
Feta cheese (crumbled)
Cherry tomatoes (halved)
Salt and pepper to taste

Preparation:
1. Sauté fresh spinach until wilted.
2. Pour whisked eggs over spinach.
3. Add crumbled feta and halved cherry tomatoes.
4. Bake until eggs are set.

Prep Time: 15 minutes
GI Value: 0 (for eggs)
GI Load: 0
Calories: ~220
Sugar Level: 2g

6. Steel-Cut Oats with Berries and Nuts

Ingredients:
Steel-cut oats
Mixed berries (blueberries, raspberries)
Nuts (walnuts, almonds)
Cinnamon and honey for flavor

Preparation:
1. Cook steel-cut oats according to package instructions.

2. Top with mixed berries, nuts, cinnamon, and a drizzle of honey.

Prep Time: 20 minutes
GI Value: 40 (approximate for steel-cut oats)
GI Load: 13
Calories: ~250
Sugar Level: 8g

7. Smoked Salmon and Cream Cheese Bagel

Ingredients:
Whole grain bagel (toasted)
Smoked salmon
Cream cheese (light or low-fat)
Capers and red onion slices

Preparation:
1. Toast a whole grain bagel.
2. Spread cream cheese on the bagel halves.
3. Top with smoked salmon, capers, and red onion slices.

Prep Time: 10 minutes
GI Value: 70 (approximate for bagel)
GI Load: 25
Calories: ~300
Sugar Level: 3g

8. Quinoa Breakfast Bowl with Fruit

Ingredients:
Quinoa (cooked)

Greek yogurt (unsweetened)
Fresh fruits (kiwi, banana, berries)
Almonds (sliced)
Drizzle of honey

Preparation:
1. Spoon cooked quinoa into a bowl.
2. Top with Greek yogurt, fresh fruits, sliced almonds, and a drizzle of honey.

Prep Time: 15 minutes (if quinoa is pre-cooked)
GI Value: 53 (approximate for quinoa)
GI Load: 13
Calories: ~300
Sugar Level: 10g

9. Low-Sugar Smoothie Bowl

Ingredients:
Mixed berries (frozen)
Spinach
Greek yogurt (unsweetened)
Chia seeds
Almond milk (unsweetened)

Preparation:
1. Blend mixed berries, spinach, Greek yogurt, chia seeds, and almond milk until smooth.
2. Pour into a bowl and add toppings like sliced almonds and chia seeds.

Prep Time: 8 minutes
GI Value: 30
GI Load: 8
Calories: ~200
Sugar Level: 8g

10. Egg and Vegetable Muffin Cups

Ingredients:
Eggs (whisked)
Bell peppers (diced)
Spinach (chopped)
Feta cheese (crumbled)
Salt and pepper to taste

Preparation:
1. Preheat the oven and grease muffin cups.
2. Mix whisked eggs with diced bell peppers, chopped spinach, crumbled feta, salt, and pepper.
3. Pour the mixture into muffin cups and bake until eggs are set.

Prep Time: 20 minutes
GI Value: 0 (for eggs)
GI Load: 0
Calories: ~150
Sugar Level: 2g

Low glycemic lunch Recipes

1. Quinoa and Vegetable Stir-Fry

Ingredients:
Quinoa (cooked)
Mixed vegetables (bell peppers, broccoli, snap peas)
Tofu or grilled chicken
Low-sodium soy sauce

Sesame oil

Garlic and ginger, minced

1. **Preparation:**
2. Stir-fry mixed vegetables, tofu or chicken, garlic, and ginger in sesame oil.
3. Add cooked quinoa and low-sodium soy sauce.
4. Toss until well combined.

Prep Time: 20 minutes

GI Value: 53 (approximate for quinoa)

GI Load: 13

Calories: ~300

Sugar Level: 3g

2. Grilled Salmon Salad

Ingredients:

Salmon fillet

Mixed greens

Cherry tomatoes

Cucumber, sliced

Balsamic vinaigrette

Olive oil

Salt and pepper to taste

Preparation:

1. Grill salmon until cooked.
2. Assemble mixed greens, cherry tomatoes, and cucumber.
3. Top with grilled salmon, drizzle with balsamic vinaigrette, and season with olive oil, salt, and pepper.

Prep Time: 15 minutes

Calories: ~350

Sugar Level: 5g

3. Mushroom and Spinach Quiche with Whole Grain Crust

Ingredients:
Whole grain pie crust
Eggs (whisked)
Mushrooms, sliced
Spinach, chopped
Feta cheese (optional)
Milk or almond milk
Salt and pepper to taste

Preparation:
1. Prebake whole grain pie crust.
2. Sauté mushrooms and spinach.
3. Whisk eggs with milk, salt, and pepper.
4. Layer sautéed vegetables and feta (if using) in the pie crust. Pour the egg mixture over.
5. Bake until the quiche is set.

Prep Time: 30 minutes
GI Value: 50 (approximate for whole grain crust)
GI Load: 20
Calories: ~250
Sugar Level: 3g

4. Turkey and Avocado Wrap

Ingredients:
Whole grain wrap
Turkey slices
Avocado, sliced
Lettuce and tomato

Greek yogurt (unsweetened)
Mustard
Salt and pepper to taste

Preparation:
Lay out the whole grain wrap.
Layer turkey slices, avocado, lettuce, and tomato.
Spread Greek yogurt and mustard, then season with
salt and pepper.
Roll into a wrap.
Prep Time: 10 minutes
GI Value: 70 (approximate for whole grain wrap)
GI Load: 25
Calories: ~300
Sugar Level: 3g

5. Lentil and Vegetable Soup

Ingredients:
Lentils
Carrots, celery, and onion (diced)
Low-sodium vegetable broth
Spinach, chopped
Cumin and coriander
Olive oil
Salt and pepper to taste

Preparation:
1. Sauté diced vegetables in olive oil until soft.
2. Add lentils, vegetable broth, cumin, coriander, salt, and pepper.
3. Simmer until lentils are cooked, then stir in chopped spinach.

Prep Time: 40 minutes

GI Value: 30 (approximate for lentils)
GI Load: 7
Calories: ~250
Sugar Level: 3g

6. Eggplant and Chickpea Salad

Ingredients:
Eggplant, cubed
Chickpeas (canned, rinsed)
Cherry tomatoes, halved
Feta cheese (optional)
Olive oil
Balsamic vinegar
Fresh basil, chopped
Salt and pepper to taste

Preparation:
1. Roast cubed eggplant until golden.
2. Combine roasted eggplant with chickpeas, cherry tomatoes, and feta.
3. Drizzle with olive oil and balsamic vinegar, then season with fresh basil, salt, and pepper.

Prep Time: 25 minutes
Calories: ~280
Sugar Level: 4g

7. Cauliflower Rice Stir-Fry

Ingredients:
Cauliflower, grated (for "rice")
Mixed vegetables (bell peppers, carrots, peas)
Shrimp or tofu
Low-sodium soy sauce

Garlic and ginger, minced
Olive oil
Green onions, chopped

Preparation:
1. Sauté mixed vegetables, shrimp or tofu, garlic, and ginger in olive oil.
2. Add grated cauliflower and cook until tender.
3. Stir in low-sodium soy sauce and garnish with chopped green onions.

Prep Time: 15 minutes
GI Value: 0 (for cauliflower)
GI Load: 0
Calories: ~250
Sugar Level: 5g

8. Chicken and Vegetable Lettuce Wraps

Ingredients:
Ground chicken
Lettuce leaves (such as iceberg or butterhead)
Mushrooms, water chestnuts, and bell peppers (chopped)
Low-sodium soy sauce
Hoisin sauce
Garlic and ginger, minced

Preparation:
1. Cook ground chicken with garlic and ginger.
2. Add chopped vegetables and stir-fry until tender.

3. Mix in low-sodium soy sauce and hoisin sauce.
4. Spoon the mixture into lettuce leaves.

Prep Time: 20 minutes
Calories: ~300
Sugar Level: 3g

9. Caprese Salad with Balsamic Glaze

Ingredients:
Tomatoes, sliced
Fresh mozzarella, sliced
Fresh basil leaves
Balsamic glaze
Olive oil
Salt and pepper to taste

Preparation:
1. Arrange tomato and mozzarella slices on a plate.
2. Tuck fresh basil leaves between slices.
3. Drizzle with balsamic glaze and olive oil. Season with salt and pepper.

Prep Time: 10 minutes
Calories: ~250
Sugar Level: 4g

10. Sweet Potato and Black Bean Bowl

Ingredients:
Sweet potatoes, cubed
Black beans (canned, rinsed)
Corn kernels
Avocado, sliced

Lime juice
Cilantro, chopped
Chili powder
Olive oil
Salt and pepper to taste

Preparation:
1. Roast sweet potatoes with chili powder, salt, and pepper until tender.
2. Combine with black beans and corn.
3. Drizzle with olive oil and lime juice, then garnish with sliced avocado and chopped cilantro.

Prep Time: 30 minutes
GI Value: 50 (approximate for sweet potatoes)
GI Load: 11
Calories: ~280
Sugar Level: 3g

Low glycemic Dinner Recipes

1. Baked Lemon Herb Chicken

Ingredients:
Chicken breasts
Fresh lemon juice
Garlic, minced
Fresh herbs (rosemary, thyme)
Olive oil
Salt and pepper to taste

Preparation:
1. Marinate chicken in lemon juice, minced garlic, fresh herbs, and olive oil.
2. Bake until chicken is cooked through.

Prep Time: 30 minutes (including marination)
Calories: ~200 per 3-ounce serving
Sugar Level: 0g

2. Salmon and Asparagus Foil Packets

Ingredients:
Salmon fillets
Asparagus spears
Lemon slices
Olive oil
Garlic, minced
Dill
Salt and pepper to taste

Preparation:
1. Place salmon fillets and asparagus on a foil sheet.
2. Drizzle with olive oil, sprinkle minced garlic, dill, salt, and pepper.
3. Seal the foil packets and bake until the salmon is flaky.

Prep Time: 25 minutes
Calories: ~250 per serving
Sugar Level: 2g

3. Vegetarian Lentil Stew

Ingredients:
Lentils
Carrots, celery, and onion (diced)
Low-sodium vegetable broth
Spinach, chopped
Cumin and coriander
Olive oil
Salt and pepper to taste

Preparation:
1. Sauté diced vegetables in olive oil until soft.
2. Add lentils, vegetable broth, cumin, coriander, salt, and pepper.
3. Simmer until lentils are cooked, then stir in chopped spinach.

Prep Time: 40 minutes
GI Value: 30 (approximate for lentils)
GI Load: 7
Calories: ~250
Sugar Level: 3g

4. Grilled Vegetable and Quinoa Stuffed Bell Peppers

Ingredients:
Bell peppers, halved
Quinoa (cooked)
Zucchini, eggplant, and tomatoes (chopped)
Feta cheese (optional)
Olive oil
Balsamic vinegar
Fresh basil, chopped
Salt and pepper to taste

Preparation:
1. Grill chopped vegetables until tender.
2. Mix grilled vegetables with cooked quinoa and feta.
3. Stuff bell peppers with the mixture.
4. Drizzle with olive oil and balsamic vinegar, then sprinkle with fresh basil, salt, and pepper.

Prep Time: 30 minutes
Calories: ~300
Sugar Level: 6g

5. Cauliflower and Chickpea Curry

Ingredients:
Cauliflower florets
Chickpeas (canned, rinsed)
Coconut milk (unsweetened)
Curry powder
Garlic and ginger, minced

Onion, diced
Olive oil
Cilantro for garnish
Salt and pepper to taste

Preparation:
1. Sauté diced onion, garlic, and ginger in olive oil until softened.
2. Add cauliflower, chickpeas, coconut milk, and curry powder. Simmer until the cauliflower is tender.
3. Season with salt and pepper, garnish with cilantro.

Prep Time: 35 minutes
Calories: ~280
Sugar Level: 4g

6. Turkey and Vegetable Skewers

Ingredients:
Turkey breast, cut into chunks
Bell peppers, cherry tomatoes, and zucchini (cut into pieces)
Olive oil
Lemon juice
Garlic, minced
Oregano
Salt and pepper to taste

Preparation:
1. Marinate turkey chunks and vegetables in olive oil, lemon juice, minced garlic, oregano, salt, and pepper.

2. Thread onto skewers and grill until turkey is
   cooked.

Prep Time: 25 minutes (including marination)
Calories: ~220 per serving
Sugar Level: 4g

7. Spaghetti Squash with Tomato and Basil Sauce

Ingredients:
Spaghetti squash
Tomatoes, diced
Fresh basil, chopped
Garlic, minced
Olive oil
Grated Parmesan cheese (optional)
Salt and pepper to taste

Preparation:
1. Roast or microwave spaghetti squash until
   tender.
2. Sauté diced tomatoes, minced garlic, and
   fresh basil in olive oil.
3. Scrape spaghetti squash strands into the pan
   and toss until well coated.
4. Season with salt and pepper. Top with grated
   Parmesan if desired.

Prep Time: 40 minutes (including
roasting/microwaving)
Calories: ~200
Sugar Level: 6g

8. Baked Cod with Lemon and Dill

Ingredients:
Cod fillets
Fresh lemon juice
Fresh dill, chopped
Garlic, minced
Olive oil
Salt and pepper to taste

Preparation:
1. Marinate cod in lemon juice, chopped dill, minced garlic, and olive oil.
2. Bake until the cod is flaky.

Prep Time: 25 minutes (including marination)
Calories: ~180 per 3-ounce serving
Sugar Level: 0g

9. Brussels Sprouts and Bacon Sauté

Ingredients:
Brussels sprouts, halved
Turkey bacon, chopped
Olive oil
Balsamic vinegar
Maple syrup (optional)
Salt and pepper to taste

Preparation:
1. Sauté halved Brussels sprouts and chopped turkey bacon in olive oil until browned.

2. Drizzle with balsamic vinegar and maple syrup (optional).
3. Season with salt and pepper.

Prep Time: 20 minutes
Calories: ~180
Sugar Level: 4g

10. Eggplant Parmesan

Ingredients:
Eggplant, sliced
Marinara sauce (low-sugar)
Mozzarella cheese, shredded
Parmesan cheese, grated
Fresh basil, chopped
Olive oil
Salt and pepper to taste

Preparation:
1. Bake or grill eggplant slices until tender.
2. Layer eggplant slices with marinara sauce, mozzarella, and Parmesan.
3. Bake until the cheese is melted and bubbly.
4. Garnish with fresh basil.

Prep Time: 40 minutes
Calories: ~250
Sugar Level: 5g

Day 1:

Breakfast: Greek Yogurt Parfait
Ingredients:
Greek yogurt (unsweetened)
Mixed berries (blueberries, strawberries)
Almonds (sliced)
Drizzle of honey (optional)

Preparation:
1. Layer Greek yogurt with mixed berries and sliced almonds.
2. Drizzle with honey if desired.

Prep Time: 5 minutes
GI Value: 30
GI Load: 6
Calories: ~200
Sugar Level: 10g

Lunch: Quinoa Salad with Grilled Chicken
Ingredients:
Quinoa (cooked)
Grilled chicken breast
Cherry tomatoes, cucumber, and bell peppers (diced)
Feta cheese (optional)
Olive oil and lemon vinaigrette

Preparation:
1. Mix cooked quinoa with diced vegetables.
2. Top with grilled chicken and feta.
3. Drizzle with olive oil and lemon vinaigrette.

Prep Time: 20 minutes

GI Value: 53 (quinoa)
GI Load: 13
Calories: ~350
Sugar Level: 5g

Dinner: Baked Lemon Herb Salmon
Ingredients:
Salmon fillets
Fresh lemon juice
Garlic, minced
Fresh herbs (rosemary, thyme)
Olive oil

Preparation:
1. Marinate salmon in lemon juice, minced garlic, and fresh herbs.
2. Bake until salmon is cooked through.

Prep Time: 30 minutes (including marination)
Calories: ~200 per 3-ounce serving
Sugar Level: 0g

Day 2:

Breakfast: Chia Seed Pudding
Ingredients:
Chia seeds
Almond milk (unsweetened)
Vanilla extract
Fresh berries for topping

Preparation:
1. Mix chia seeds with almond milk and vanilla extract.
2. Refrigerate until the pudding thickens.

3. Top with fresh berries before serving.

Prep Time: 5 minutes (+ chilling time)

GI Value: 1

GI Load: 0

Calories: ~150

Sugar Level: 1g

Lunch: Lentil and Vegetable Soup

Ingredients:

Lentils

Carrots, celery, and onion (diced)

Low-sodium vegetable broth

Spinach, chopped

Cumin and coriander

Olive oil

Preparation:

1. Sauté diced vegetables in olive oil until soft.
2. Add lentils, vegetable broth, cumin, coriander, salt, and pepper.
3. Simmer until lentils are cooked, then stir in chopped spinach.

Prep Time: 40 minutes

GI Value: 30 (lentils)

GI Load: 7

Calories: ~250

Sugar Level: 3g

Dinner: Grilled Vegetable and Quinoa Stuffed Bell Peppers

Ingredients:

Bell peppers, halved

Quinoa (cooked)

Zucchini, eggplant, and tomatoes (chopped)
Feta cheese (optional)
Olive oil
Balsamic vinegar
Fresh basil, chopped

Preparation:
1. Grill chopped vegetables until tender.
2. Mix grilled vegetables with cooked quinoa and feta.
3. Stuff bell peppers with the mixture.
4. Drizzle with olive oil and balsamic vinegar, then sprinkle with fresh basil, salt, and pepper.

Prep Time: 30 minutes
Calories: ~300
Sugar Level: 6g

Day 3:

Breakfast: Avocado and Tomato Omelette
Ingredients:
Eggs (whisked)
Avocado (sliced)
Cherry tomatoes (halved)
Fresh basil (chopped)

Preparation:
1. Make an omelette with whisked eggs.
2. Fill with sliced avocado, cherry tomatoes, and fresh basil.
3. Season with salt and pepper.

Prep Time: 10 minutes
GI Value: 0 (eggs)

GI Load: 0
Calories: ~250
Sugar Level: 2g

Lunch: Turkey and Vegetable Skewers
Ingredients:
Turkey breast, cut into chunks
Bell peppers, cherry tomatoes, and zucchini (cut into pieces)
Olive oil
Lemon juice
Garlic, minced
Oregano

Preparation:
1. Marinate turkey chunks and vegetables in olive oil, lemon juice, minced garlic, oregano, salt, and pepper.
2. Thread onto skewers and grill until turkey is cooked.

Prep Time: 25 minutes (including marination)
Calories: ~220 per serving
Sugar Level: 4g

Dinner: Cauliflower and Chickpea Curry
Ingredients:
Cauliflower florets
Chickpeas (canned, rinsed)
Coconut milk (unsweetened)
Curry powder
Garlic and ginger, minced
Onion, diced
Olive oil

Cilantro for garnish

Preparation:
1. Sauté diced onion, garlic, and ginger in olive oil until softened.
2. Add cauliflower, chickpeas, coconut milk, and curry powder. Simmer until the cauliflower is tender.
3. Season with salt and pepper, garnish with cilantro.

Prep Time: 35 minutes
Calories: ~280
Sugar Level: 4g

Day 4:

Breakfast: Whole Grain Toast with Smashed Avocado
Ingredients:
Whole grain bread (toasted)
Avocado (smashed)
Cherry tomatoes (sliced)

Preparation:
1. Toast whole grain bread.
2. Spread smashed avocado on the toast.
3. Top with sliced cherry tomatoes and season with sea salt and black pepper.

Prep Time: 7 minutes
GI Value: 30 (approximate for whole grain bread)
GI Load: 10
Calories: ~200
Sugar Level: 2g

Lunch: Brussels Sprouts and Bacon Sauté
Ingredients:
Brussels sprouts, halved
Turkey bacon, chopped
Olive oil
Balsamic vinegar
Maple syrup (optional)

Preparation:
1. Sauté halved Brussels sprouts and chopped turkey bacon in olive oil until browned.
2. Drizzle with balsamic vinegar and maple syrup (optional).
3. Season with salt and pepper.

Prep Time: 20 minutes
Calories: ~180
Sugar Level: 4g

Dinner: Spaghetti Squash with Tomato and Basil Sauce
Ingredients:
Spaghetti squash
Tomatoes, diced
Fresh basil, chopped
Garlic, minced
Olive oil
Grated Parmesan cheese (optional)

Preparation:
1. Roast or microwave spaghetti squash until tender.
2. Sauté diced tomatoes, minced garlic, and fresh basil in olive oil.

3. Scrape spaghetti squash strands into the pan and toss until well coated.
4. Season with salt and pepper. Top with grated Parmesan if desired.

Prep Time: 40 minutes (including roasting/microwaving)
Calories: ~200
Sugar Level: 6g

Day 5:

Breakfast: Berry and Spinach Smoothie
Ingredients:
Mixed berries (blueberries, strawberries)
Spinach leaves
Greek yogurt (unsweetened)
Almond milk (unsweetened)
Chia seeds

Preparation:
Blend mixed berries, spinach, Greek yogurt, almond milk, and chia seeds until smooth.
Prep Time: 7 minutes
GI Value: Varies (dependent on berries)
GI Load: Varies
Calories: ~250
Sugar Level: 10g

Lunch: Eggplant and Chickpea Salad
Ingredients:
Eggplant, cubed
Chickpeas (canned, rinsed)
Cherry tomatoes, halved
Feta cheese (optional)

Olive oil
Balsamic vinegar
Fresh basil, chopped

Preparation:
1. Roast cubed eggplant until golden.
2. Combine roasted eggplant with chickpeas, cherry tomatoes, and feta.
3. Drizzle with olive oil and balsamic vinegar, then season with fresh basil, salt, and pepper.

Prep Time: 25 minutes
Calories: ~280
Sugar Level: 4g

Dinner: Baked Cod with Lemon and Dill
Ingredients:
Cod fillets
Fresh lemon juice
Fresh dill, chopped
Garlic, minced
Olive oil

Preparation:
1. Marinate cod in lemon juice, chopped dill, minced garlic, and olive oil.
2. Bake until the cod is flaky.

Prep Time: 25 minutes (including marination)
Calories: ~180 per 3-ounce serving
Sugar Level: 0g

Day 6:

Breakfast: Oatmeal with Berries and Nuts
Ingredients:
Rolled oats
Mixed berries (blueberries, raspberries)
Almonds, chopped
Almond milk (unsweetened)
Cinnamon

Preparation:
1. Cook rolled oats with almond milk until creamy.
2. Top with mixed berries, chopped almonds, and a sprinkle of cinnamon.

Prep Time: 10 minutes
GI Value: 55 (rolled oats)
GI Load: 13
Calories: ~250
Sugar Level: 6g

Lunch: Caprese Salad with Balsamic Glaze
Ingredients:
Tomatoes, sliced
Fresh mozzarella, sliced
Fresh basil leaves
Balsamic glaze
Olive oil

Preparation:
1. Arrange tomato and mozzarella slices on a plate.
2. Tuck fresh basil leaves between slices.

3. Drizzle with balsamic glaze and olive oil. Season with salt and pepper.

Prep Time: 10 minutes
Calories: ~250
Sugar Level: 4g

Dinner: Turkey and Avocado Wrap

Ingredients:
Whole grain wrap
Turkey slices
Avocado, sliced
Lettuce and tomato
Greek yogurt (unsweetened)
Mustard

Preparation:

1. Lay out the whole grain wrap.
2. Layer turkey slices, avocado, lettuce, and tomato.
3. Spread Greek yogurt and mustard, then season with salt and pepper.
4. Roll into a wrap.

Prep Time: 10 minutes
GI Value: 70 (approximate for whole grain wrap)
GI Load: 25
Calories: ~300
Sugar Level: 3g

Day 7:

Breakfast: Sweet Potato and Black Bean Bowl

Ingredients:
Sweet potatoes, cubed
Black beans (canned, rinsed)

Corn kernels
Avocado, sliced
Lime juice
Cilantro, chopped
Chili powder

Preparation:
1. Roast sweet potatoes with chili powder, salt, and pepper until tender.
2. Combine with black beans and corn.
3. Drizzle with olive oil and lime juice, then garnish with sliced avocado and chopped cilantro.

Prep Time: 30 minutes
GI Value: 50 (approximate for sweet potatoes)
GI Load: 11
Calories: ~280
Sugar Level: 3g

Lunch: Chicken and Vegetable Lettuce Wraps
Ingredients:
Ground chicken
Lettuce leaves (such as iceberg or butterhead)
Mushrooms, water chestnuts, and bell peppers (chopped)
Low-sodium soy sauce
Hoisin sauce
Garlic and ginger, minced

Preparation:
1. Cook ground chicken with garlic and ginger.
2. Add chopped vegetables and stir-fry until tender.

3. Mix in low-sodium soy sauce and hoisin sauce.
4. Spoon the mixture into lettuce leaves.

Prep Time: 20 minutes
Calories: ~300
Sugar Level: 3g

Dinner: Eggplant Parmesan

Ingredients:
Eggplant, sliced
Marinara sauce (low-sugar)
Mozzarella cheese, shredded
Parmesan cheese, grated
Fresh basil, chopped

Preparation:

1. Bake or grill eggplant slices until tender.
2. Layer eggplant slices with marinara sauce, mozzarella, and Parmesan.
3. Bake until the cheese is melted.

prep Time: 30 minutes

CONCLUSION

As we close the pages of the "Seniors' Low Glycemic Index Diet Cookbook 2024: Nourishing Your Health with Smart Choices," we sincerely hope this culinary journey has been both enlightening and delectable. Through these carefully curated recipes, we aimed not only to tantalize your taste buds but also to empower you with the knowledge and tools to make health-conscious choices that resonate with your unique nutritional needs.

Embracing a low glycemic index lifestyle is not just about managing blood sugar; it's a holistic approach to nurturing your well-being. By choosing whole, nutrient-dense foods and crafting meals with a focus on the glycemic index, you've taken a significant step towards fostering stable energy levels, supporting heart health, and promoting cognitive function.

Remember, this cookbook is not just a collection of recipes; it's a celebration of the joy that can be found in nourishing your body with purpose. As you continue on this path, savoring each bite of these wholesome dishes, we encourage you to explore and personalize, making these recipes your own.

Your health journey is unique, and the choices you make in the kitchen can contribute profoundly to your vitality. As we part ways, we want to express our deepest gratitude for allowing us to be a part of your culinary adventure. May these recipes continue to bring joy to your table, and may your health flourish with each mindful bite.

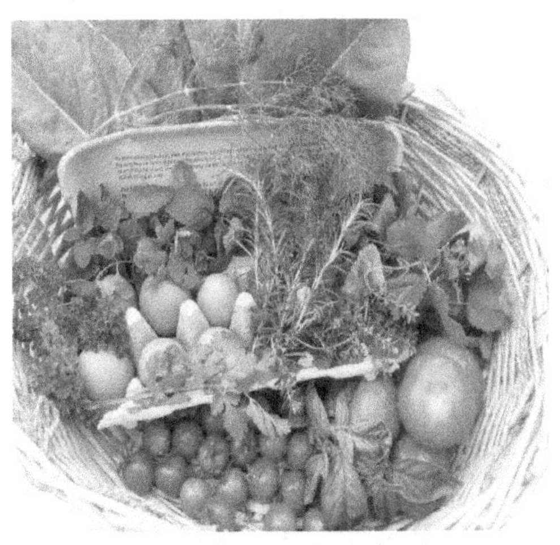

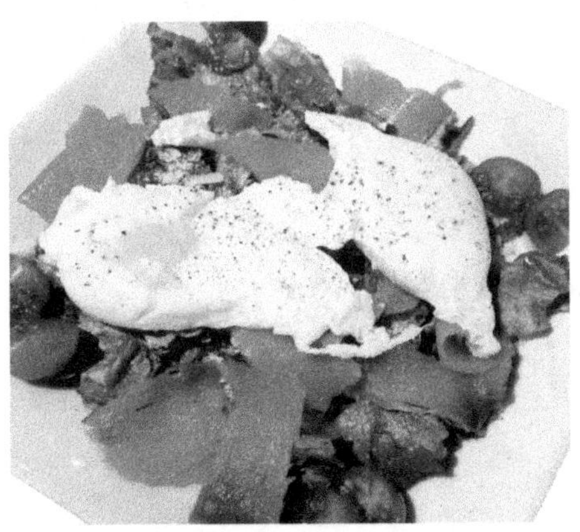